Les Techniques
Danielle Gagné

Zapping
Self-Love

Coloring Book 2

Self-Aware and
Self-Respect Exercises
in the Kitchen
and at Work

Design and Layout: MJ Schwader

Editor: MJ Schwader

Copyright © 2017 by Danielle Gagné

ISBN-13: 978-1973810599
ISBN-10: 197381059X

Dedication

To my beloved mother Mireille Gagné, to whom I offer all the honor of this book.

Acknowledgments

Stylist Linda Morisset: Designer Les Productions Linda Morisset.

Consultant Nikkea B Devida: Expert on accelerated results.

Writing Coach MJ Schwader: Editor, Design and Layout of Cover and Interior.

Sourcing LinkedIn Thérèse Lever: Psychologist en Libérale.

Director of Studies Professor Malcolm LeGrice: Supervisor of my research on Self-Analysis and the Arts at Central St Martins, University of the Arts London, who encouraged me to write a book and become a lecturer at University.

Dr. Yves Lamontagne for introducing me to Professor Isaac Marks at Maudsley Hospital, part of the Academic Health Science Centre, affiliated with King's College in London, England.

Professor Isaac Marks, who gave me the opportunity to observe and study Behavioural Therapy at Maudsley Hospital, London.

To Jean-Paul Sylvain, a Montréal journalist covering my television work at Télé-Métropole and Radio-Canada, and Terry Tighe, a photographer in London who supported and photographed my research at University. Each of you encouraged and inspired me for my 25-year mission to develop the Zapping therapy as an incredible tool for my followers.

To my husband, Dr. Paul Lelliott, psychiatrist extraordinaire, thank you for all of your support and love.

To Andrée Gagné, social worker, for being my sister.

Zapping Self-Love Coloring Book 2

Contents

Color Your Way to Deeper Transformation

This coloring book illustrates the Zapping Self-Love, Self-Care, and Shiatsu exercises that I've described in more detail in my book, *Zapping: Your Body at Your Service*, and my eBooks, Coloring Books, and e-Coloring Books. By coloring the images, you activate three senses that deepen the transformation you will have from doing the exercises. These three senses are vision, touch, and hearing:

- Vision: Seeing or imagining images of you and others helps create a picture in your mind of what you want to change.

- Touch: Coloring activates a physical response.

- Hearing: Saying affirmations while coloring will integrate the energy into your being.

Each image has a brief description of what to do and say while coloring the parts of the body. The images are of the author doing the described activity; while doing the exercises, imagine that it is *your* body you are coloring. Filling in the white spaces of the clothing will integrate the information more deeply into your own body.

There may be times when you are not able to physically color the images. When that is the case, you can use a method called "magnetic coloring" to embody in your mind the changes in the exercises that will have a powerful effect. The most significant symbol in each image is the heart. The connection with your heart is the direct link to your brain. By focusing your vision on the hearts in each image, then doing the affirmations and exercises, you can closely simulate the benefits that coloring the images will have.

Zapping refers to a specific position of cupping the hand to access your energetic field for information, combined with clockwise and counterclockwise rotation when using acupressure (based on the Shiatsu self-routine called "Do In"), visualization, and affirmations designed to shift the energy. Your Zapping hand is like a magic wand, your communication access into your inner body. It is the link between your senses and the immediate experience of visualization and affirmation. Your hand in this cupped-hand position transforms you back to your initial state of calmness at a phenomenally fast rate by decluttering unwanted energy and restoring it with self-esteem and self-love.

Color Yourself Smiling/Self-Love

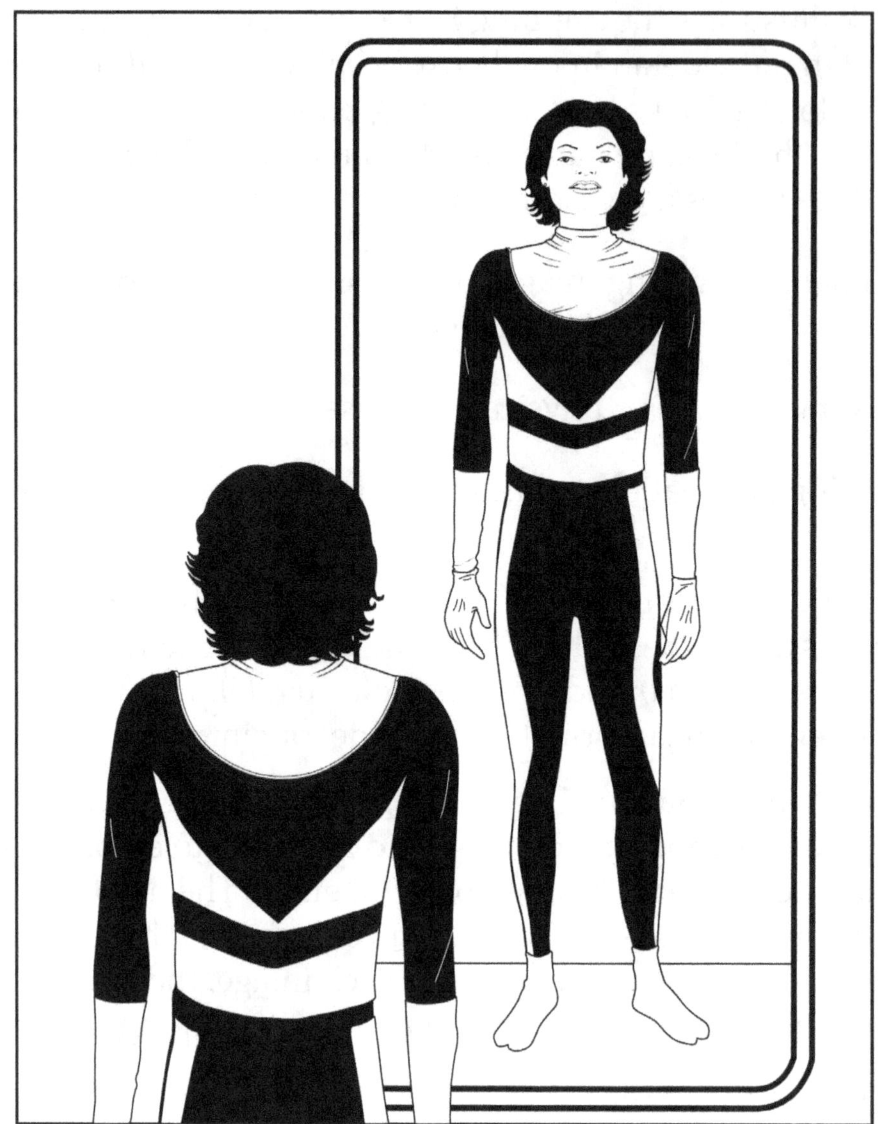

Figure 2.1 – Color Yourself Smiling/Self-Love

Color yourself acknowledging yourself in the mirror with a smile and a positive outlook. An ultimate self-care practice is to accept yourself with gentleness. Make sure you start the day with a smile, whether you are looking in the mirror or not. Repeat several times during the day ☺.

Color Yourself Decluttering and Zapping in Self-Love During the Day

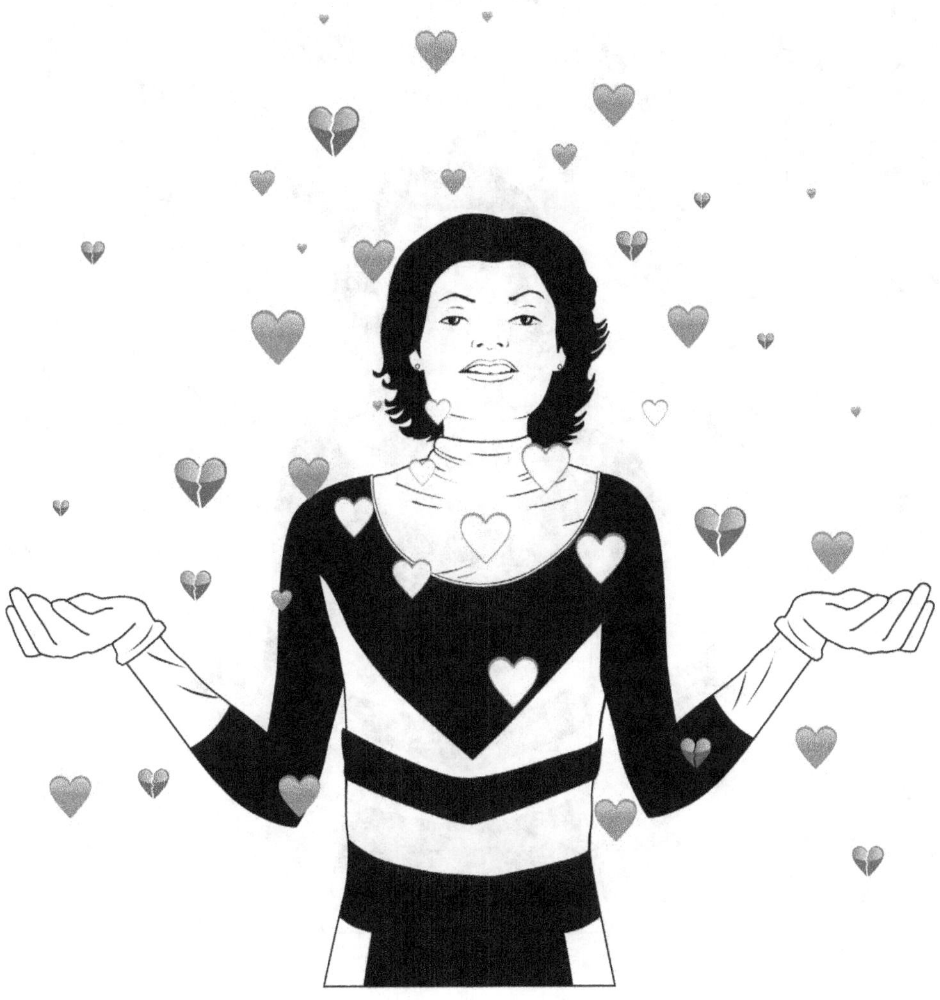

Figure 2.2 – Color Yourself Decluttering and Zapping in Self-Love During the Day

The white hearts in the figure above represent the feeling of emptiness you might experience. Allow yourself a moment to feel grounded and to have your sense of self-love restored as you color in those hearts.

Declutter your energy while focusing with intention on fully loving yourself. Being mentally and physically healthy allows you to consistently give love to the dear ones in your life.

Color Yourself with Heart Pieces that are Calm and Flowing

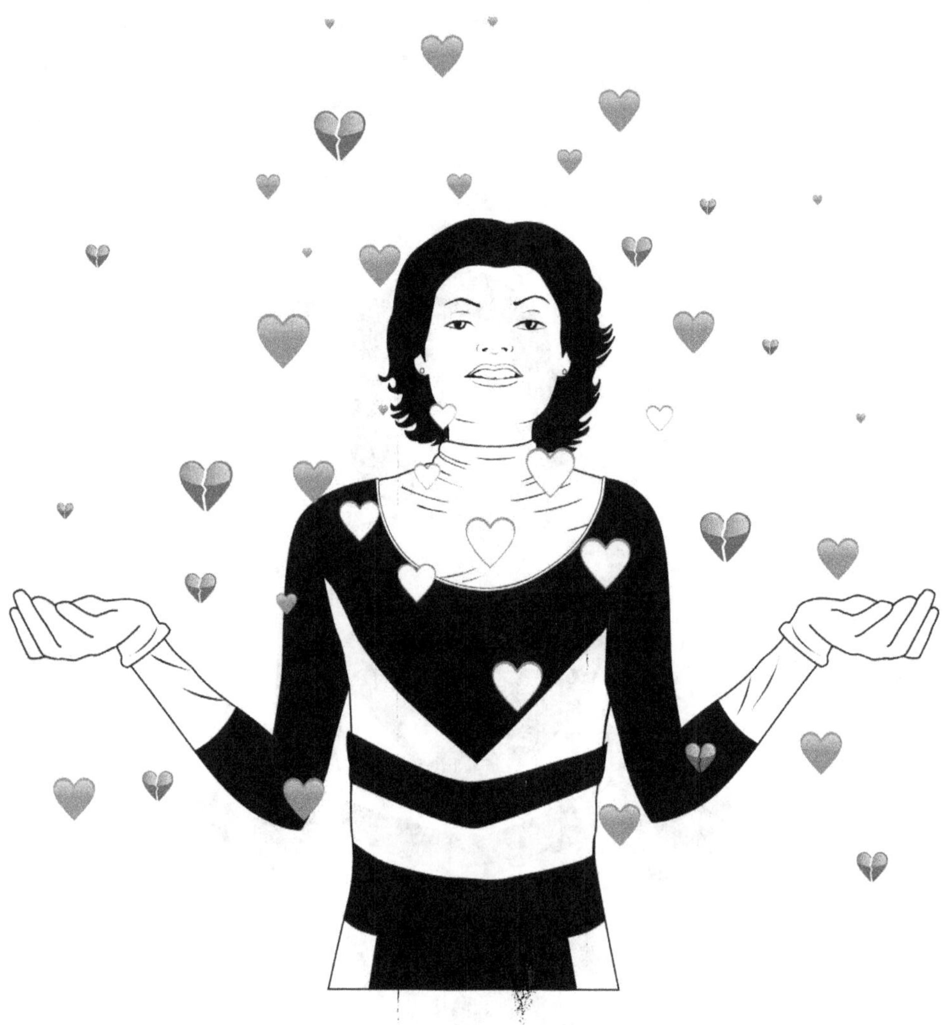

*Figure 2.3 – Color Yourself with Heart Pieces that are
Calm and Flowing*

Color the hearts in Figure 2.3 while imagining that all of the beautiful red hearts are radiating fully in a calm body that is flowing smoothly. In that state of body and mind, say the following: "I feel and enjoy my heart energy free from outside influences and energy. I focus on my self-care."

Take a deep breath. Maintain your visualization and continue the affirmation: "I am the consolidator of my heart. I am self-aware and focused on my self-care."

Color Yourself with "I Am My Own Body's Buddy" in Your Daily Activities

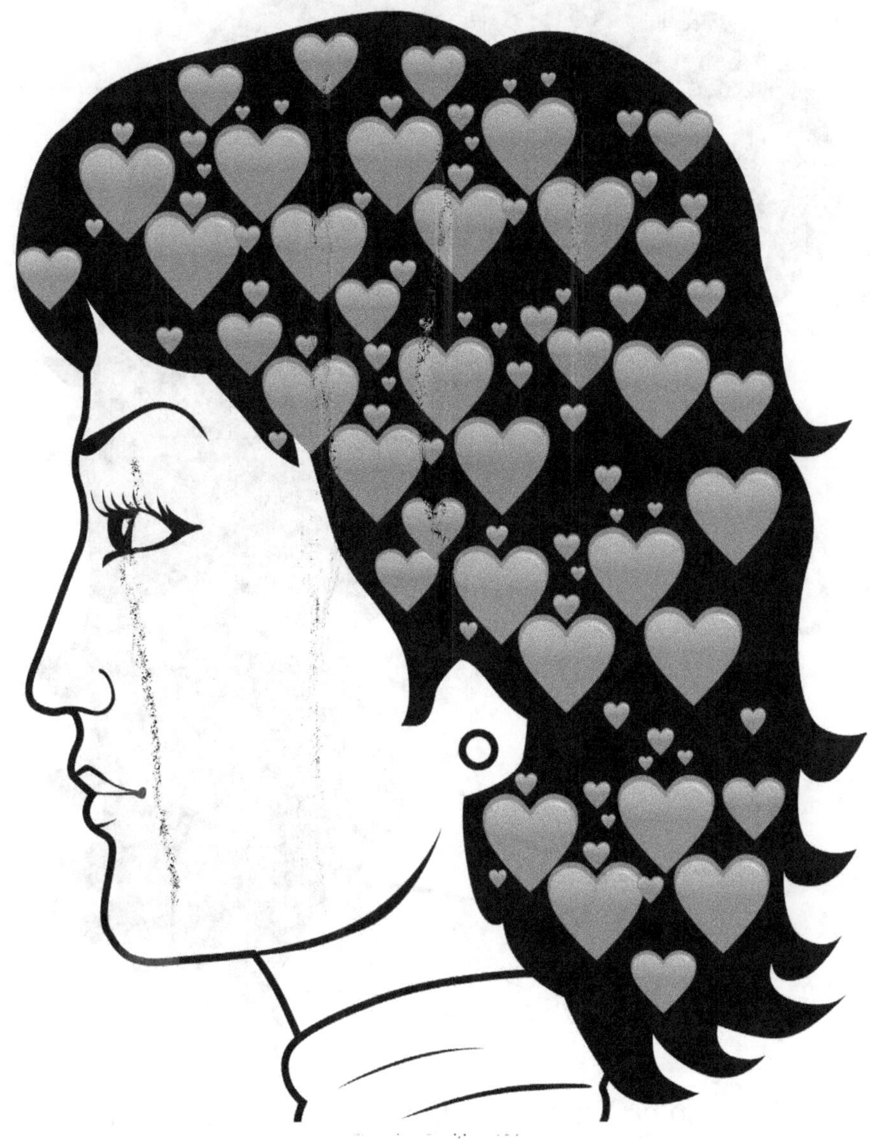

Figure 2.4 – Color Yourself with
"I Am My Own Body's Buddy" in Your Daily Activities

Color yourself imagining your head full of self-love red hearts, as you say the following: "I am my own body's buddy." Remember to do this visualization during the day as you are walking, or when you are looking at yourself in the mirror. Doing this every day brings awareness and focus on what you think and desire.

Color Yourself Going Out Being Filled with Self-Love

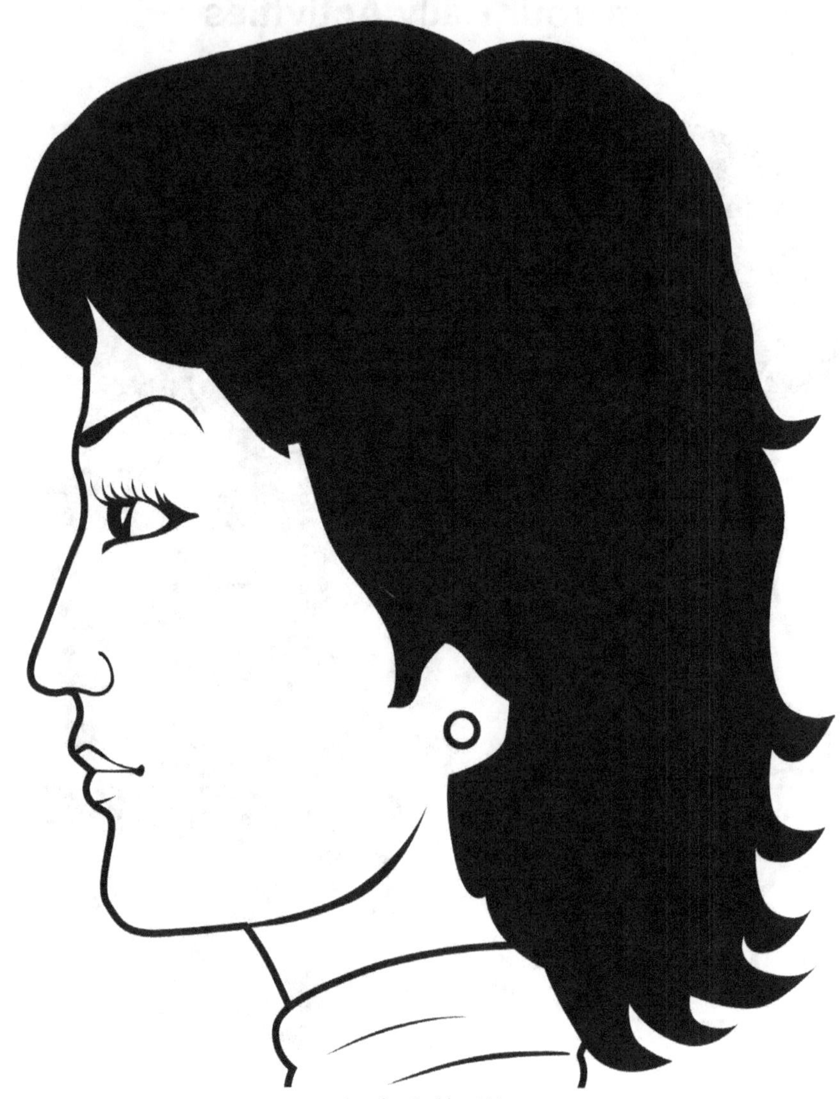

Figure 2.5 – Color Yourself Going Out Being Filled with Self-Love

You are the protector of your precious body and the energy that nourishes your mind and body. When you go out into the world, you are like an ambassador, filling your inner self with love while helping others. Coloring this exercise helps you be more aware of and deeply connected with your inner, protecting self. By filling your body with self-loving energy, you are respecting who you are and taking responsibility for how you show up in the world.

Color Yourself Sending Love Energy Back to Mother

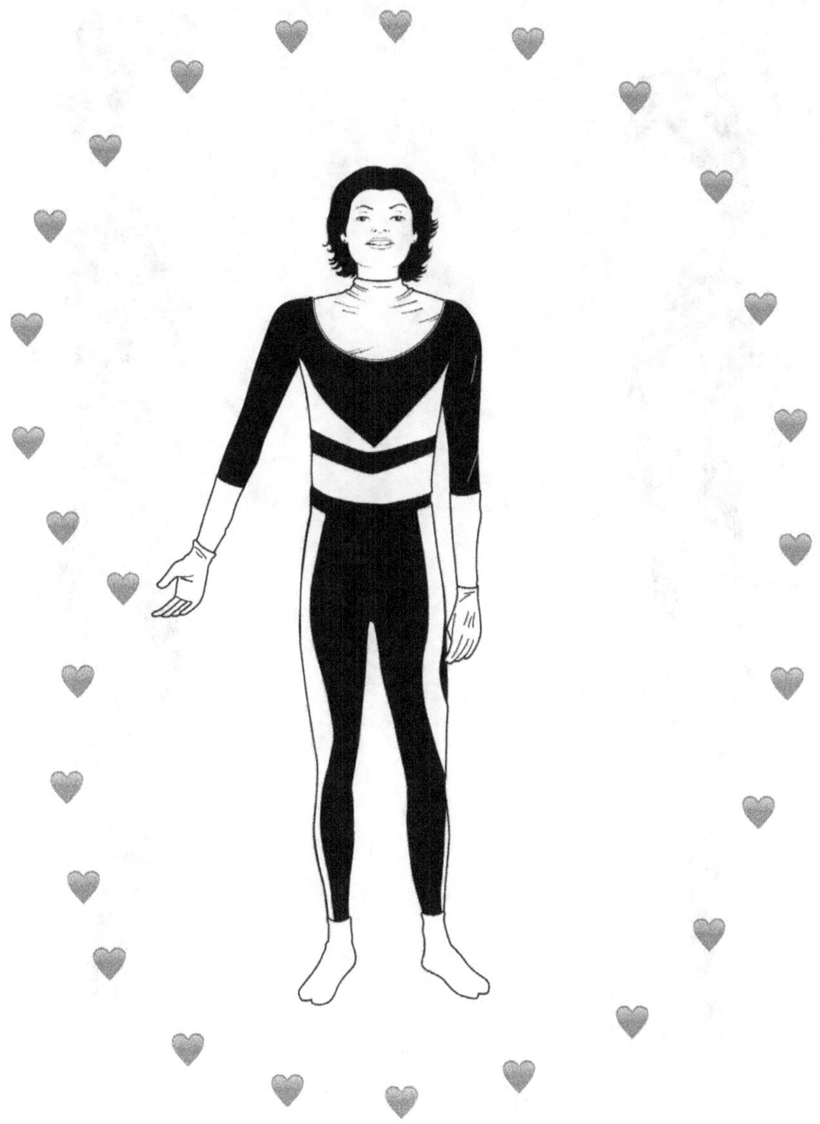

Figure 2.6 – Color Yourself Sending Love Energy Back to Mother

Color yourself waving your hand upward in a circle, visualizing a wheel of hearts, then back to the initial position, all the time focusing on sending love to your mother.

Color Yourself Sending Love Back to Another Person

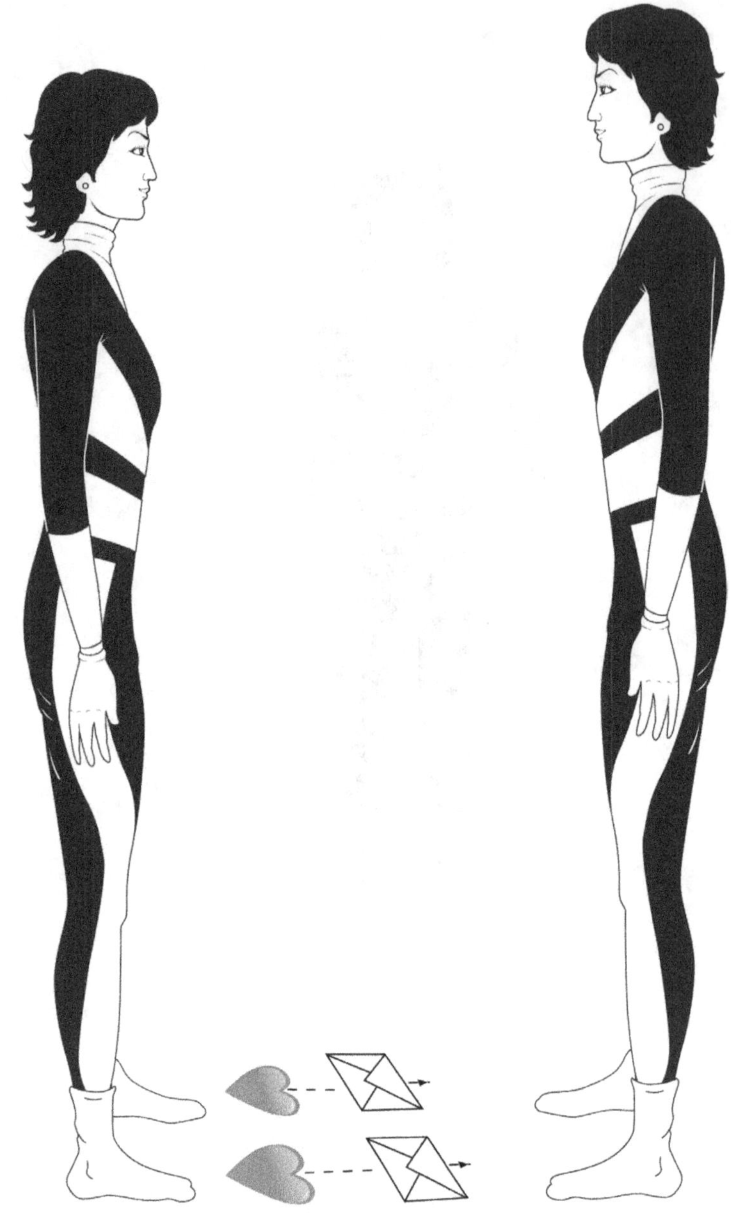

Figure 2.7 – Color Yourself Sending Love Back to Another Person

Color Figure 2.7 as you visualize envelopes on the floor with hearts on them and an arrow pointing towards the other person. With confidence, send the person love in your visualization.

Color Yourself Finding Discomfort in Your Body
Before Brushing Your Teeth

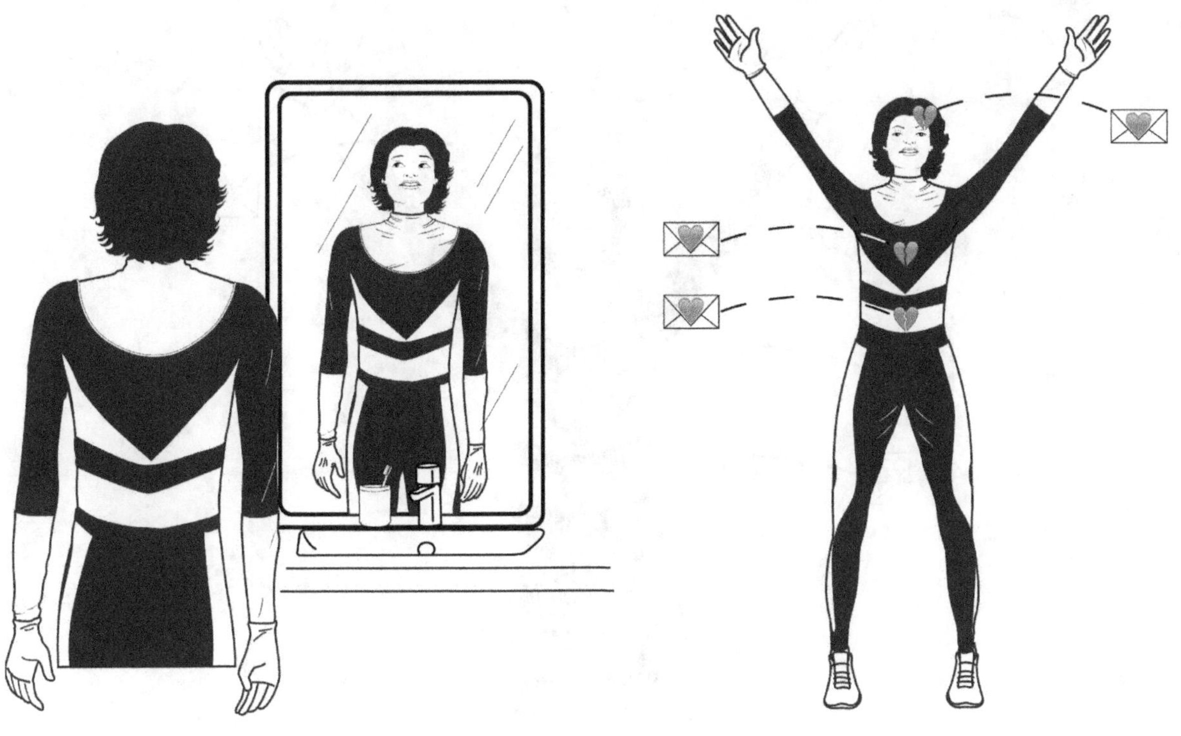

Figure 2.8 – Color Yourself Finding Discomfort in Your Body Before Brushing Your Teeth

The best place to declutter your energy is before you brush your teeth every morning. When you do this, you will be sending back broken hearts that do not belong to you.

Color yourself looking into the mirror as you visualize where in your body you are feeling discomfort. Then color Figure 2.9 on the next page as you continue with the affirmation.

Color Yourself with "I Declutter My Energy Before I Start the Day" Affirmation Every Morning Before Brushing Your Teeth

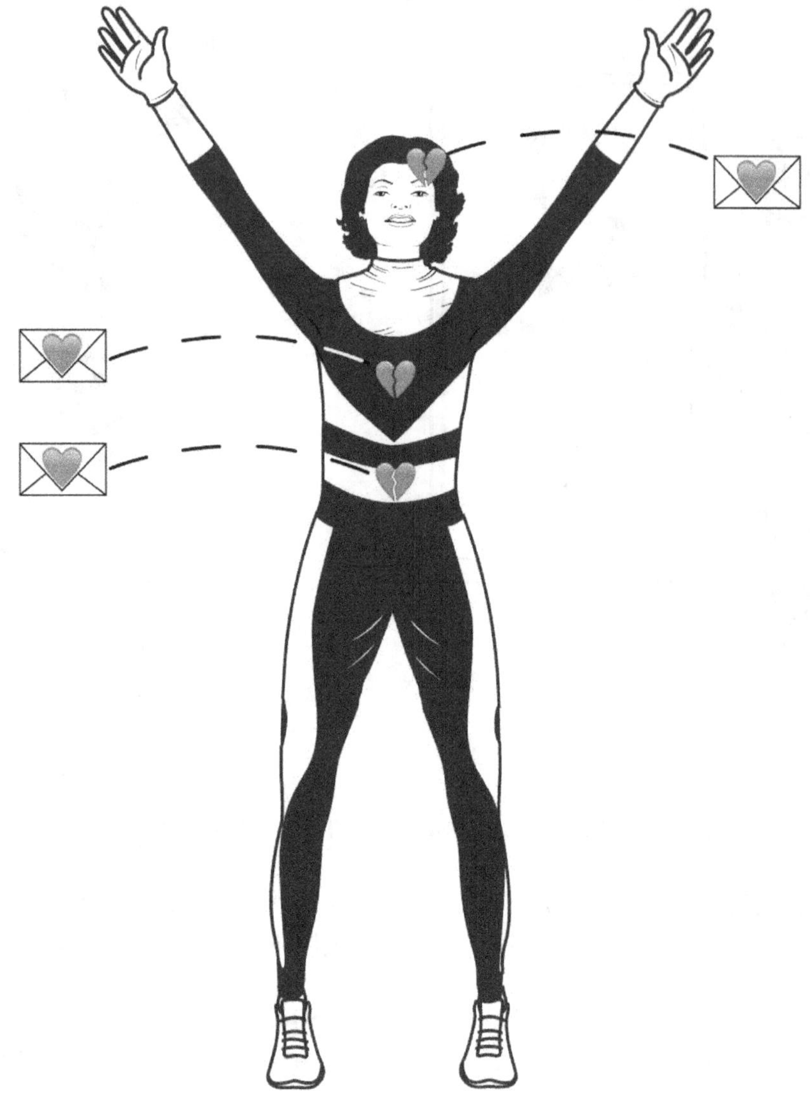

Figure 2.9 – Color Yourself with "I Declutter My Energy Before I Start the Day" Affirmation Every Morning Before Brushing Your Teeth

Color sending the energy of love back to whatever or whoever gave you discomfort. Imagine decluttering your energy, as you say, "I declutter my energy before I start the day." Imagine looking at yourself in the mirror, brushing your teeth, and starting the day.

Color Yourself Before Dressing

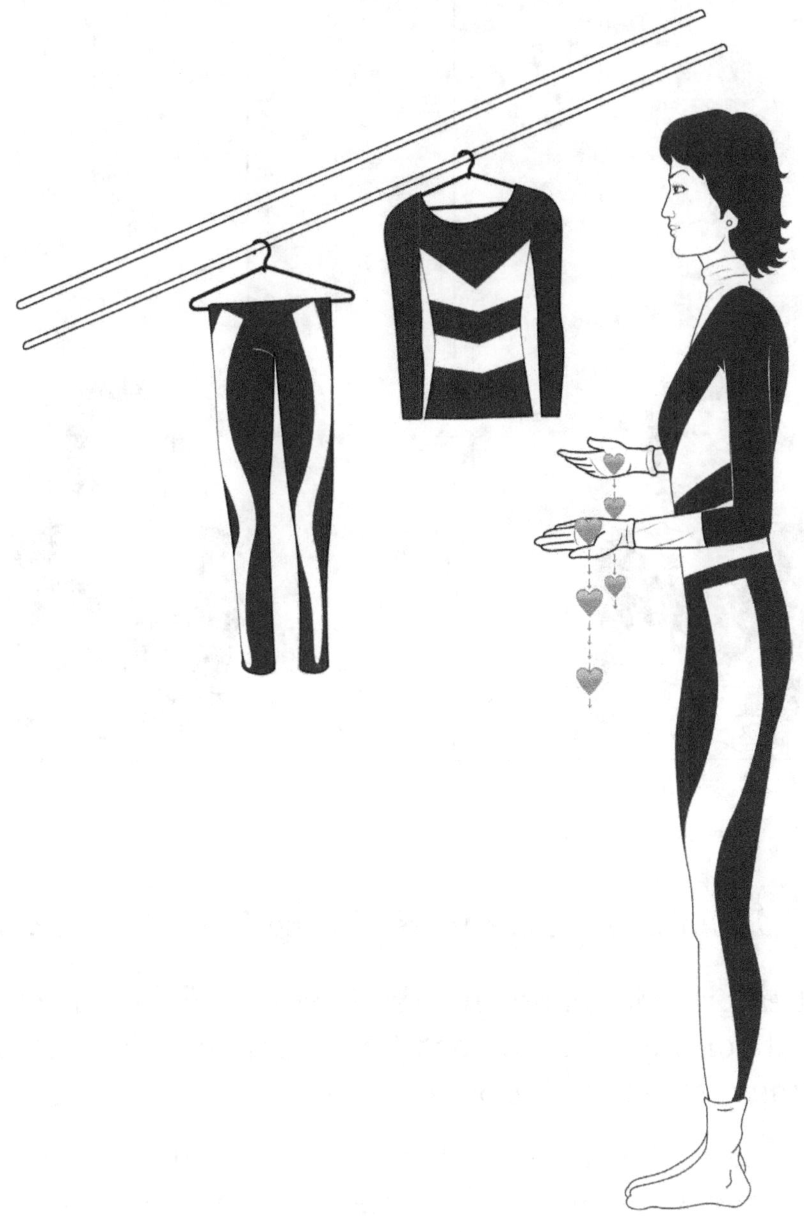

Figure 2.10 – Color Yourself Before Dressing

Imagine yourself before dressing in the morning, while your clothes are still hanging in the wardrobe, and visualize choosing what you are going to wear. Now picture a row of three red hearts on each side of your hands. Color Figure 2.10 with self-love and calmness.

Color Yourself Being Grounded at Work

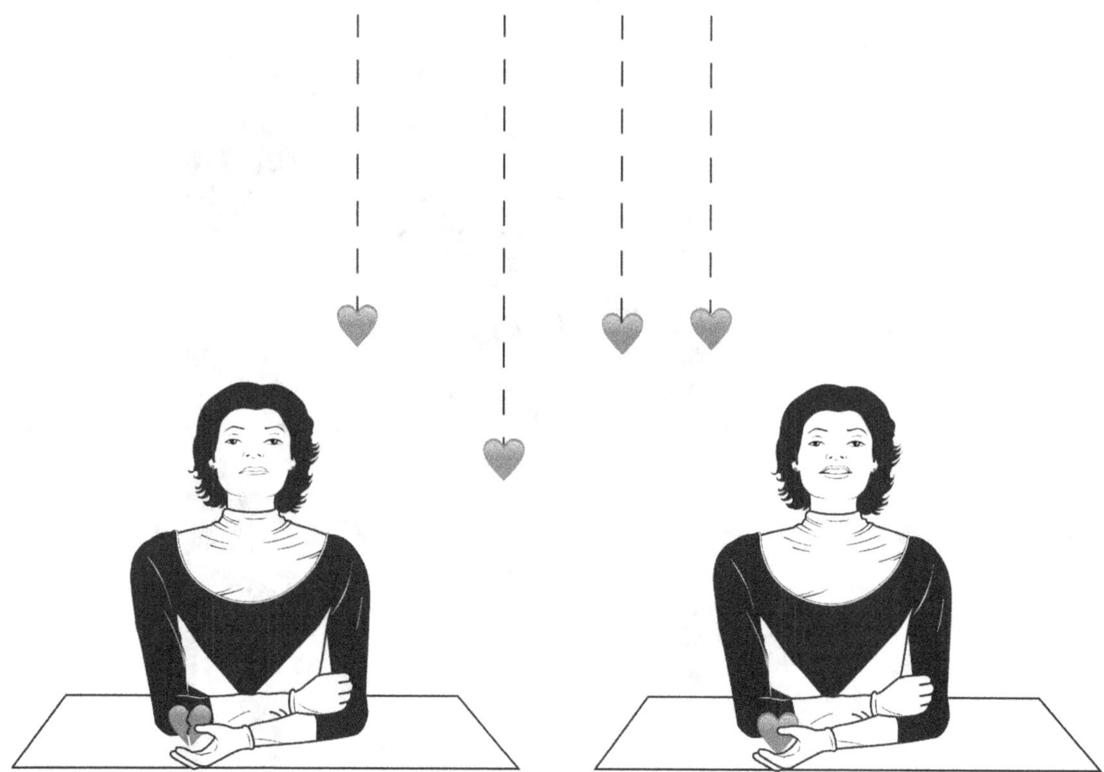

Figure 2.11 – Color Yourself Being Grounded at Work

Imagine a broken heart in your hand and a sad expression on your face. Next, imagine yourself smiling and holding a full red heart in your hand. Coloring this exercise gives you an instant feeling of peace and groundedness.

Smiling to yourself every two hours during the day declutters your feeling of emptiness and sends away the broken, sad energy. By doing these smiling exercises, you own your true healthy energy of self-love. Zapping your energy is a priority for a calm and grounded life.

Color Yourself in the Kitchen Loving Yourself
by Preparing Good, Healthy Food

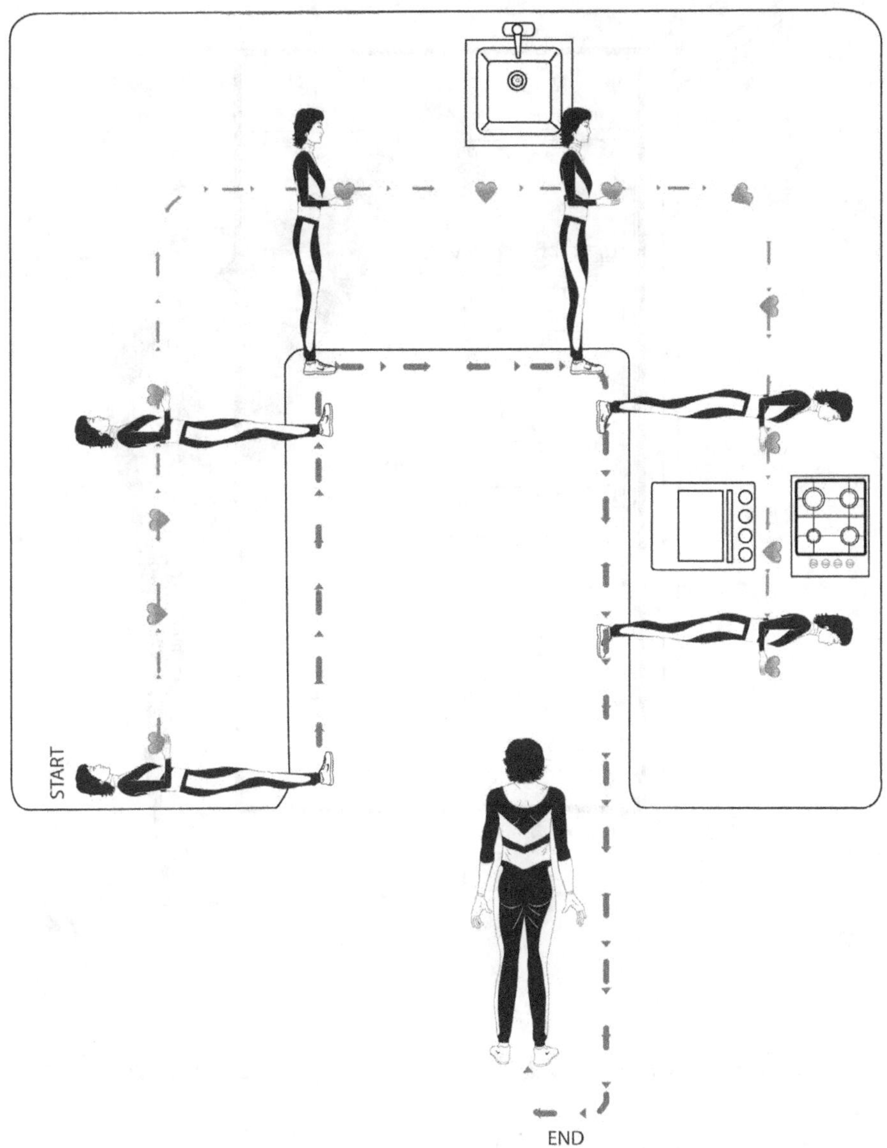

*Figure 2.12 – Color Yourself in the Kitchen Loving Yourself
by Preparing Good, Healthy Food*

Color yourself taking a self-love walk through your kitchen with a red heart in your hand, as shown in Figure 2.12. Imagine looking around the kitchen after the walk and saying to yourself, "I love myself." Now you are ready to start cooking with self-love.

Color Yourself Before Taking Food from the Refrigerator

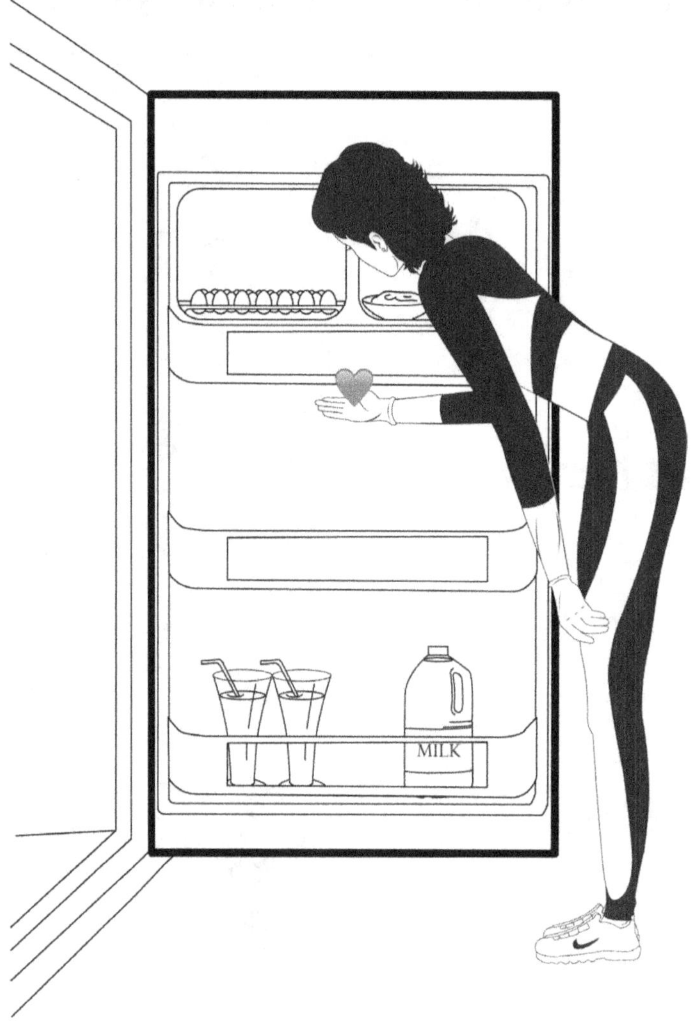

Figure 2.13 – Color Yourself Before Taking Food from the Refrigerator

Color yourself looking at your food with the image of a heart in your hand, as you quietly say to yourself, "I love and accept myself. Anything I choose from the fridge is a type of love for myself. I am sending self-love to myself by choosing it, cooking it, and eating it. I am a strong person and grounded. I am good and kind to myself. I invest time for my body because it is my best buddy."

Color Yourself Reassuring Your Inner Child

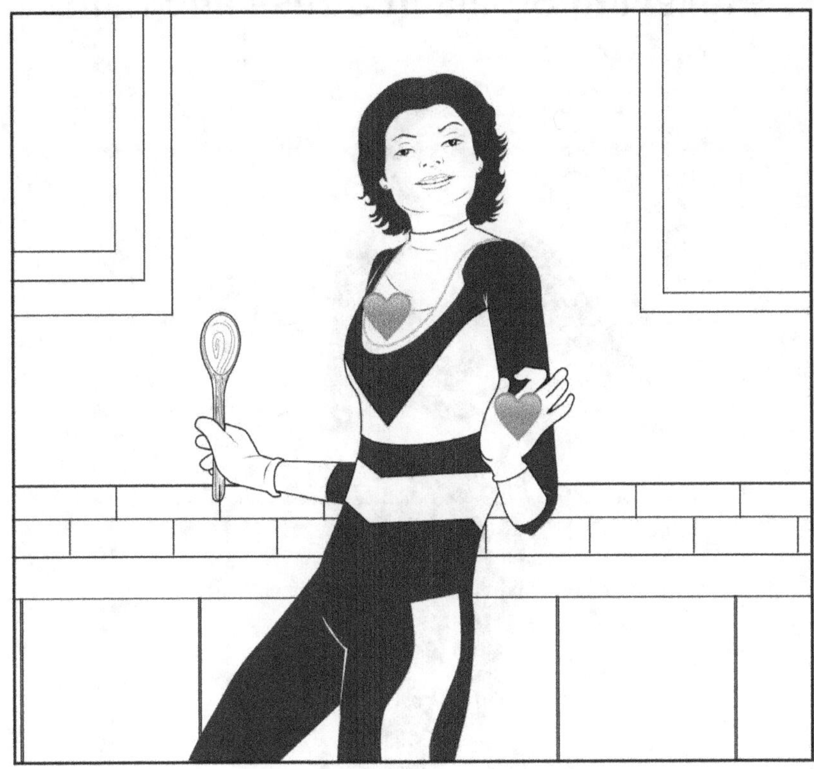

Figure 2.14 – Color Yourself Reassuring Your Inner Child

Color Figure 2.14 as you say the following to your inner child: "Do not feel abandoned [your name]. I am here for you. You have a beautiful heart and are a very nice person. You are not alone. I am here for you 100%. Come and eat with me as I cook for us. We will feel nourished with good, healthy food, enjoying our time reminiscing together. What happened was not your fault. The people who criticized or abandoned you did not know better at the time. They did the best they knew at that stage in their life. As we take expansive breaths together, know that I love you."

Color Zapping Kindness with Thumb Stroke: Relieving Stomach Stress and Pain

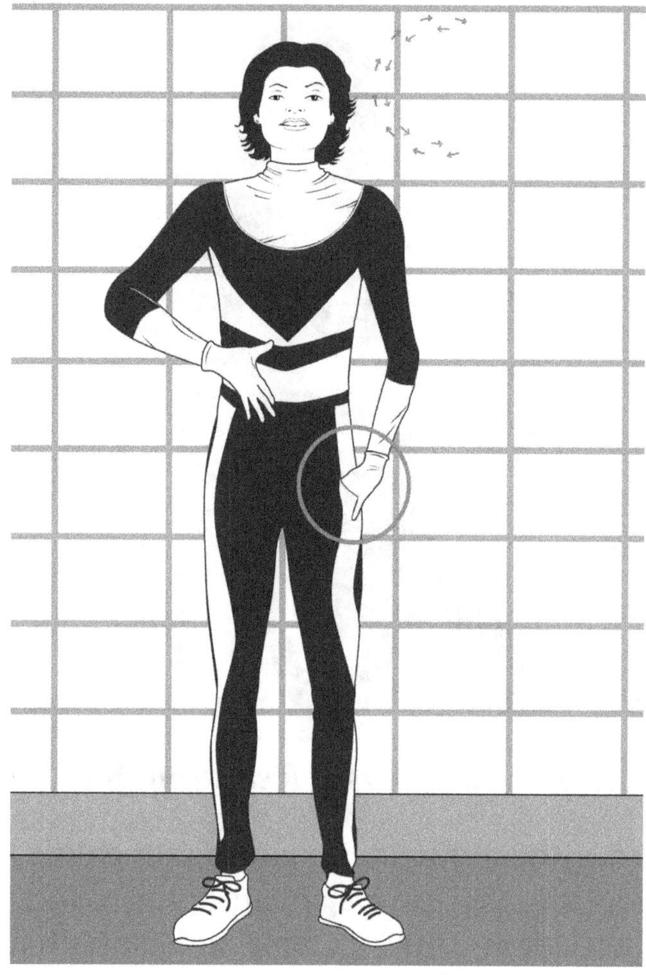

Figure 2.15 – Color Yourself Zapping Kindness with Thumb Stroke: Relieving Stomach Stress and Pain

The Zapping Shiatsu Stroking point is one of the most popular points when using Zapping Shiatsu. In particular, it zaps stress and relieves pain in the stomach. Color yourself standing and stroking your stomach with your thumb, first clockwise as shown in Figure 2.15 above, then counter-clockwise.

Color Yourself with the Power of Your Hand – Right Side

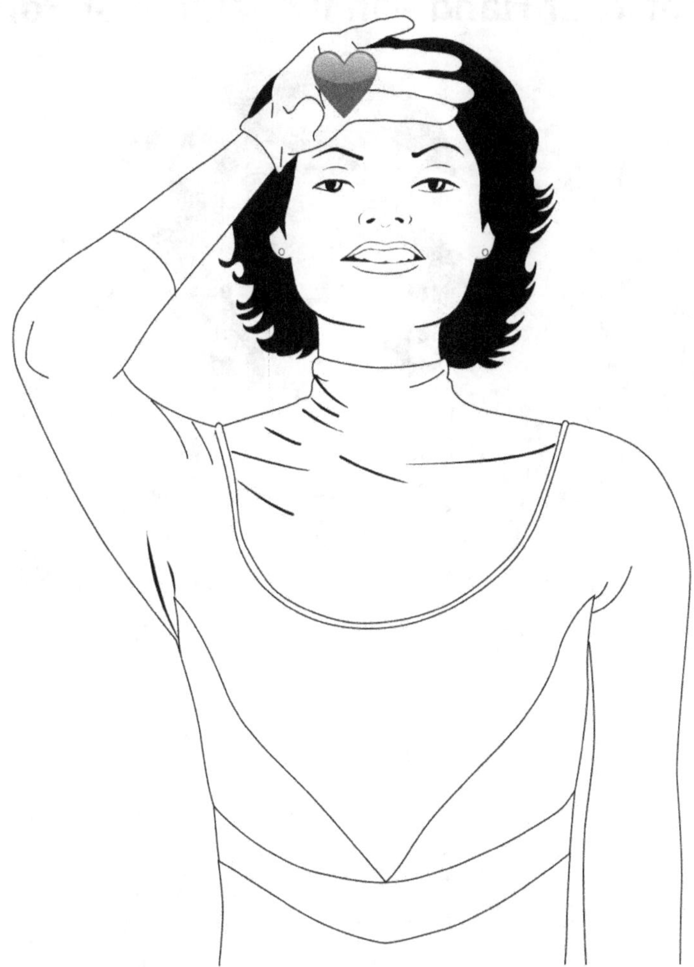

*Figure 2.16 – Color Yourself with the
Power of Your Hand – Right Side*

Color yourself placing the back side of your right hand on the right side of your forehead. Visualize a red heart in the middle of your hand.

Say the following affirmation: "I am caring for the well-being of my body. My body is my best companion; it might be with me for 100 years. I respect it; I do not endanger it. Thank you for being there for me every moment of my life. I love you, body." Take a fresh breath and take a moment to acknowledge your gratitude.

Figures 2.16, 2.17, and 2.18 are done as a sequence to be more conscious in your body.

Color Yourself with the
Power of Your Hand – in the Middle of Forehead

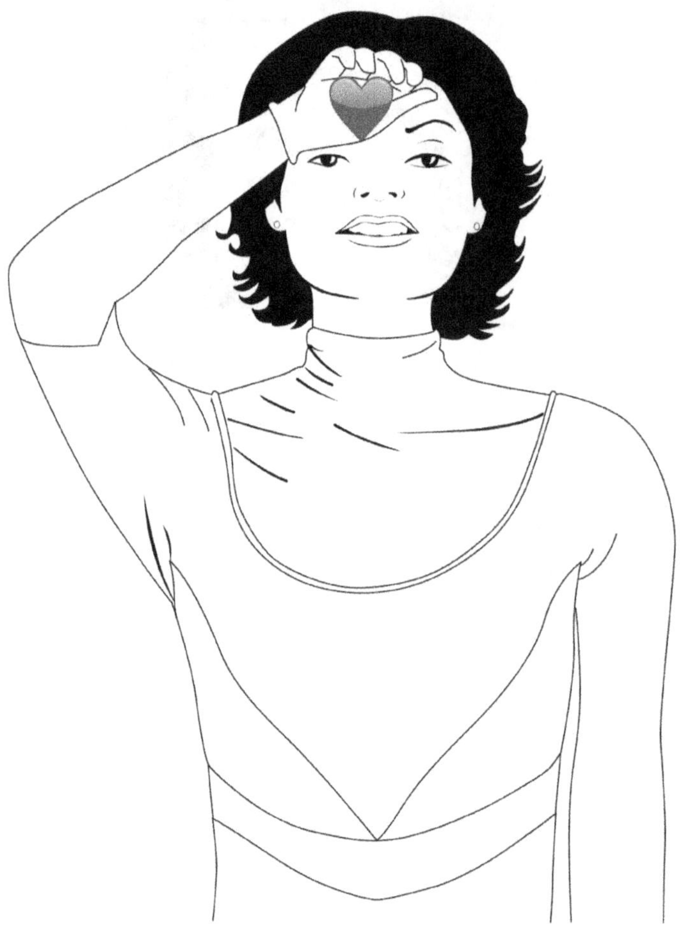

Figure 2.17 – Color Yourself with the
Power of Your Hand – in the Middle of Forehead

Color yourself raising the back of your right hand to the middle of your forehead (see Figure 2.17). Visualize a red heart in the middle of your hand.

As you color, say the following affirmation: "I love my health. I do the best for it." Imagine keeping your hand in that position for 20 seconds. Take a fresh breath and acknowledge your gratitude, then continue with Figure 2.18.

Color Yourself with the Power of Your Hand - Left Side

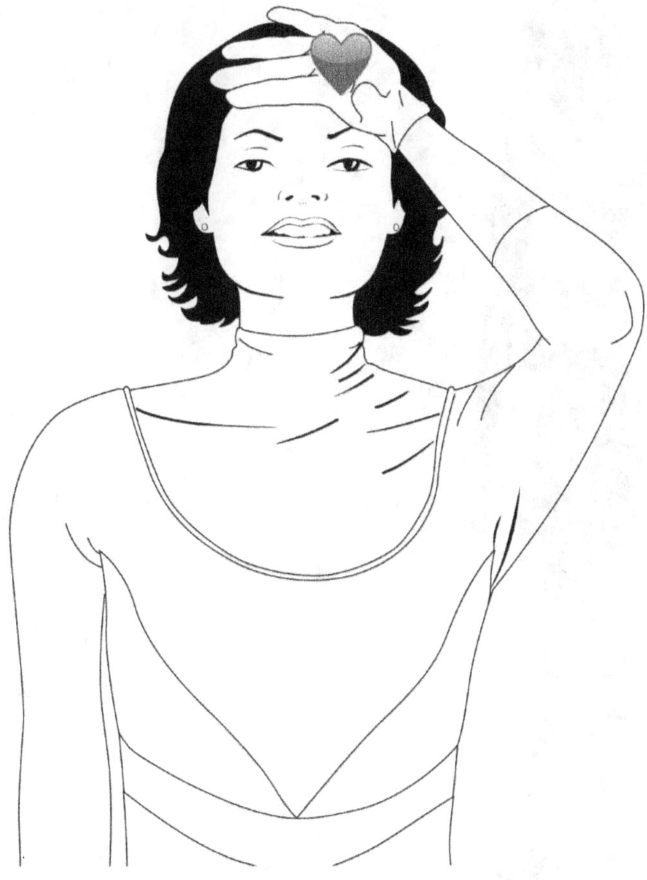

Figure 2.18 – Color Yourself with the
Power of Your Hand – Left Side

Start with becoming present in your body. Color yourself placing the back of your left hand on the left side of your forehead with your eyes looking forward. Taking a fresh breath, say the following affirmation: "I like to feed my body well. I take time to eat and chew well." Take a fresh breath and add the following: "It is the perfect time to relax when I eat. I do not force my body to swallow quickly. I enjoy chewing my food." Take a fresh breath, and express your gratitude to your body.

Color Yourself with Natural Food from Nature

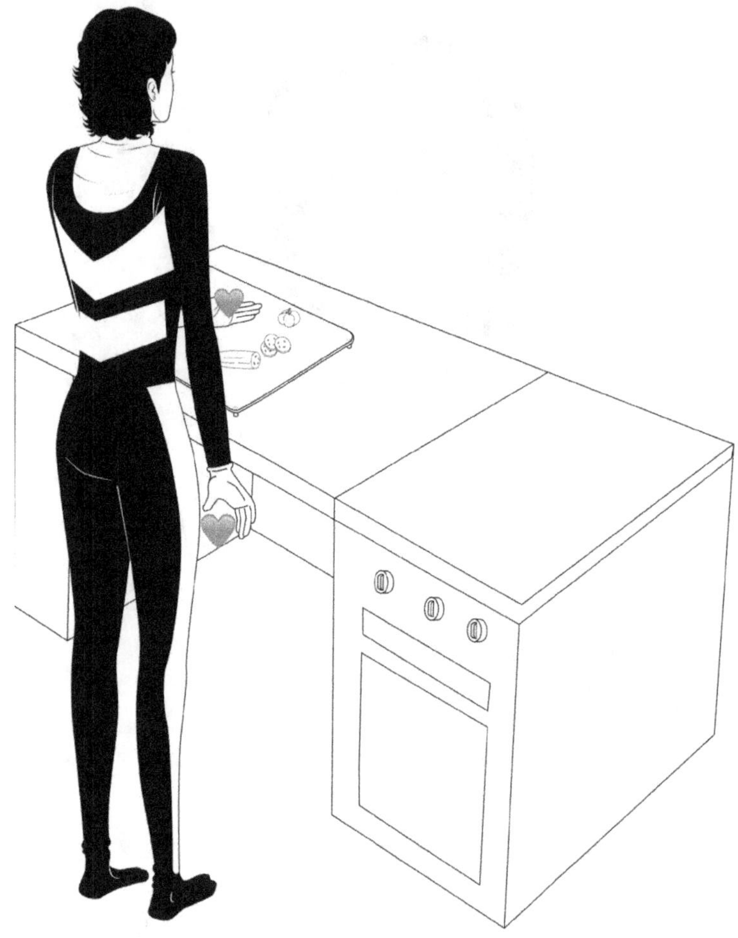

*Figure 2.19 – Color Yourself with
Natural Food from Nature*

What you eat and digest brings vital energy to your body. Eating whole organic foods whenever possible provides the self-care and protection of your body that truly reflects being of service to yourself. The key is to buy and eat foods that are full of pure energy, avoiding processed foods that irritate your body. The earlier in life you change to healthy eating habits, the better your body will feel decade after decade.

The combination of filling your body with self-love and natural food will give you a feeling of wholeness and calm, reflecting a healthy individual who shines from inside out.

Color yourself in the kitchen with natural food from nature.

Color Yourself Day-Dreaming

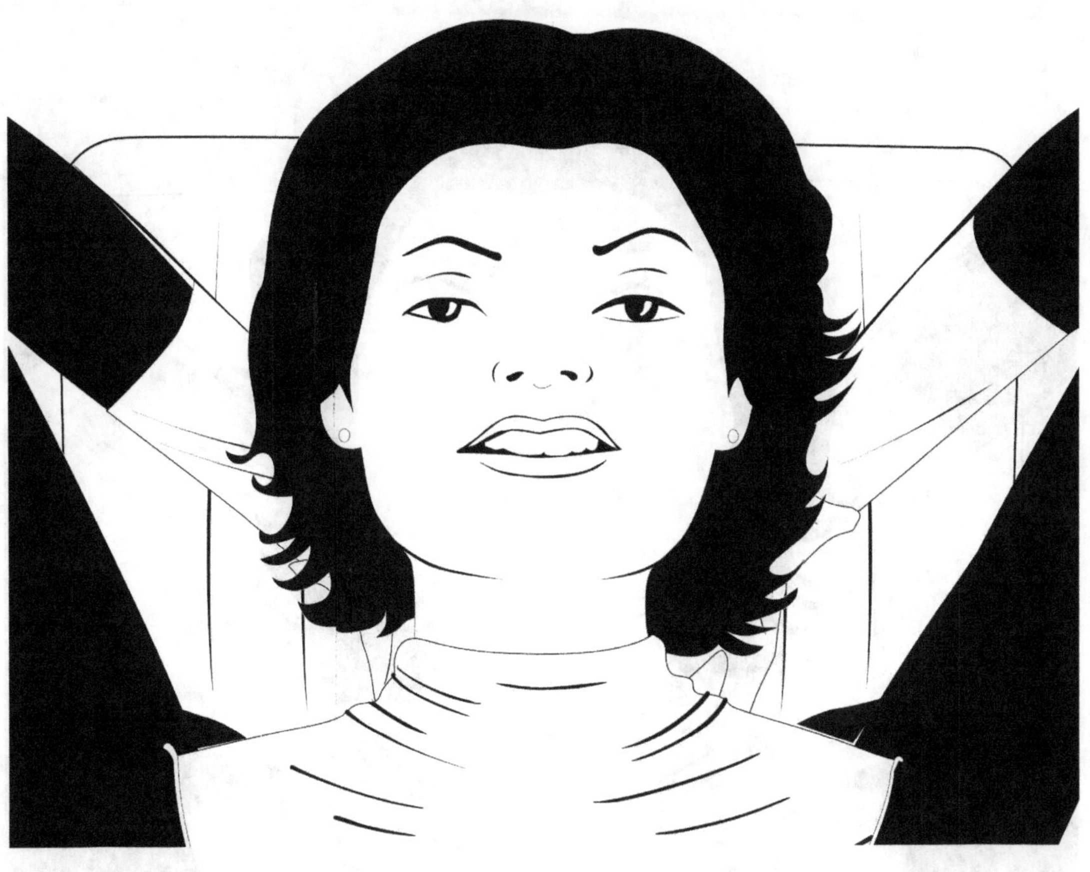

Figure 2.20 – Color Yourself Day-Dreaming

You are the manager of your body. When you listen to what it's telling you, you will thrive. Day-dreaming builds an image for what you want to manifest, and by acting on the good feelings it creates in your body, you begin to bring what you want to your life.

Color yourself day-dreaming as you say the affirmation: "Day-dreaming brings me self-awareness and images of what to manifest and what to let go to thrive."

Color Yourself Dreaming a Visualization that Connects the Higher Self Deep Within Your Body

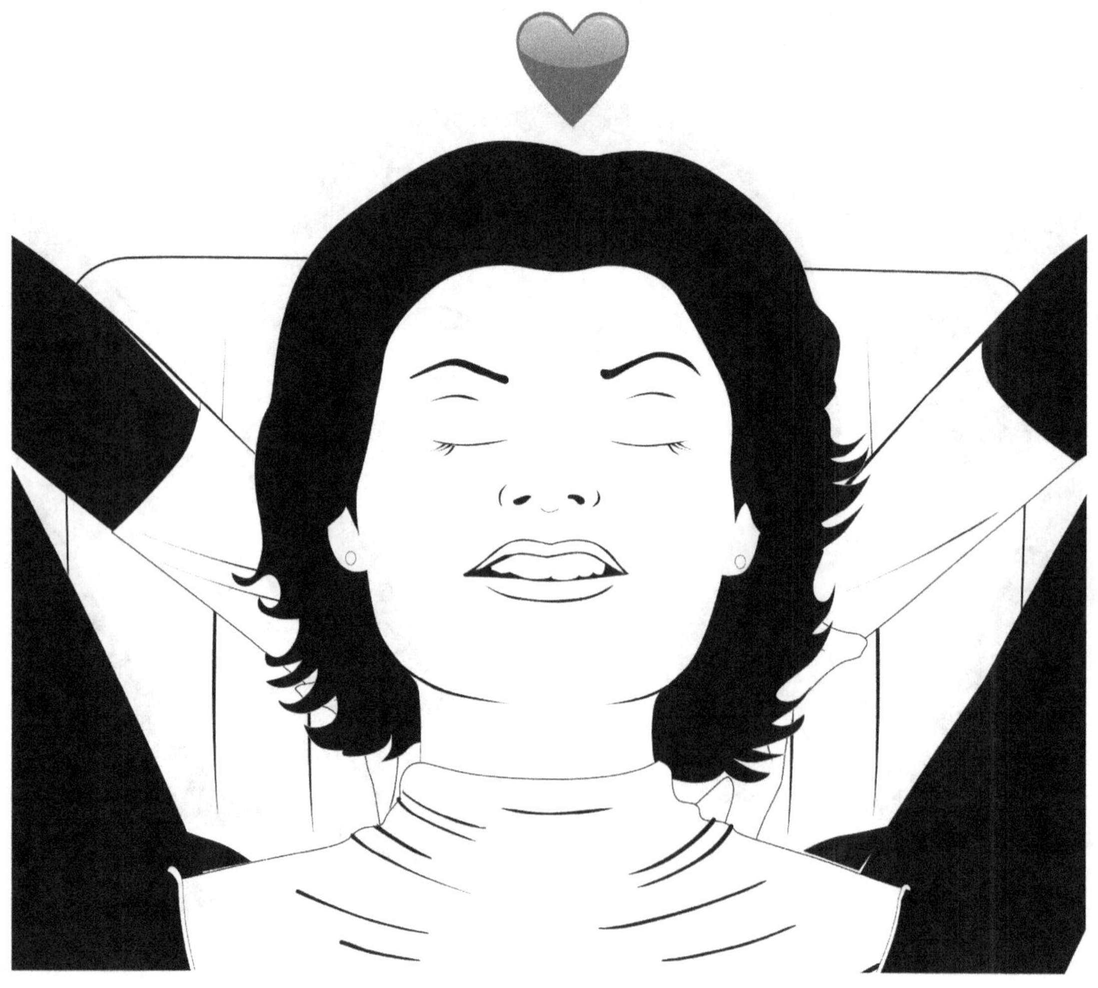

Figure 2.21 – Color Yourself Dreaming a Visualization that Connects the Higher Self Deep Within Your Body

Your inner connection to yourself brings a higher level of self-care so you can live a healthy and fulfilling life free of unwanted cluttered energy that can bring your energy down.

Color yourself connecting to the higher self to create a deep healing within your body.

Color Yourself with Complete Self-Respect

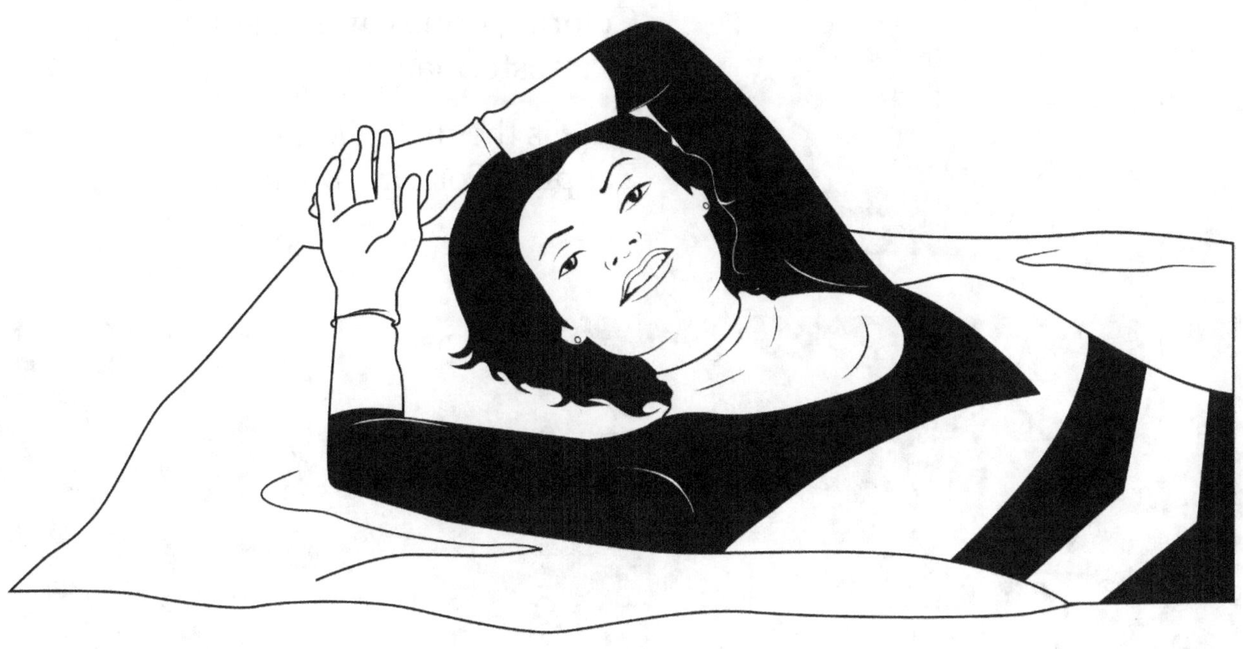

Figure 2.22 – Color Yourself with Complete Self-Respect

Imagine lying on your back and anchoring the presence of your body, as in Figure 2.22. You are the master of your body. This beautiful energy results in a calm and fulfilled life. Color you feeling self-respect.

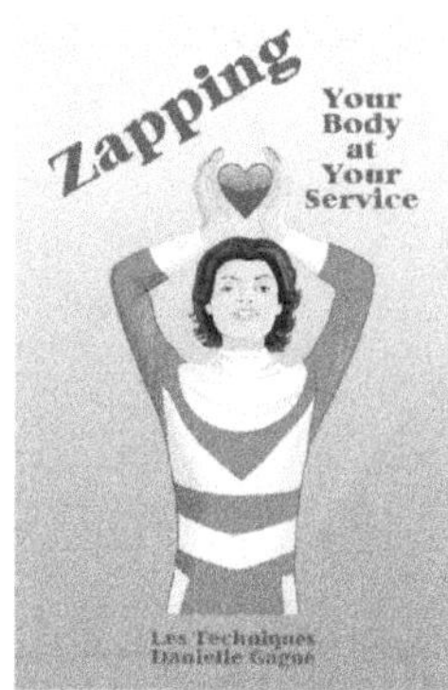

Your Body is Precious!

Coloring brings awareness to its transformation.

Here is the full collection of Zapping Coloring Books…

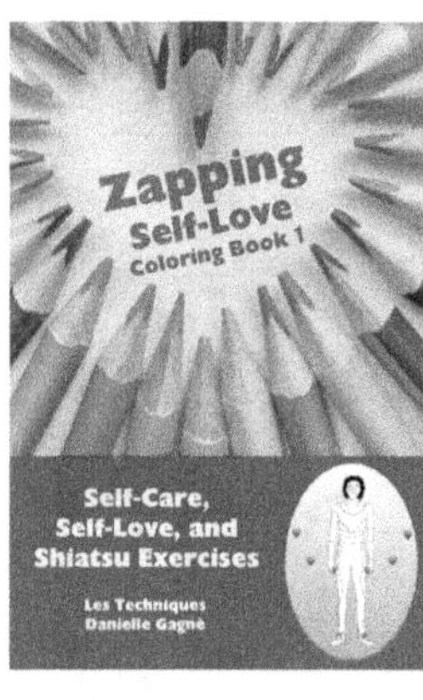
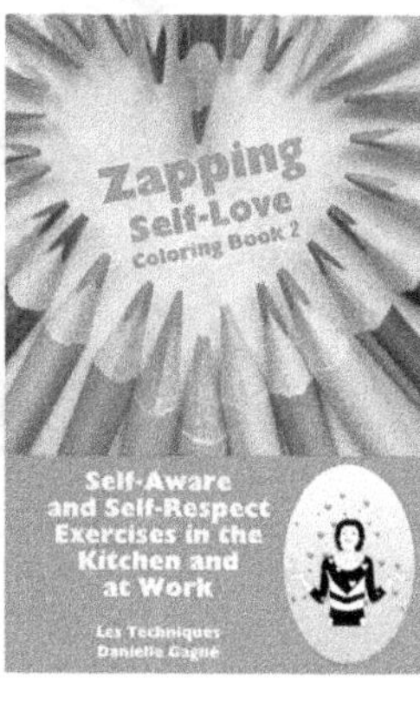
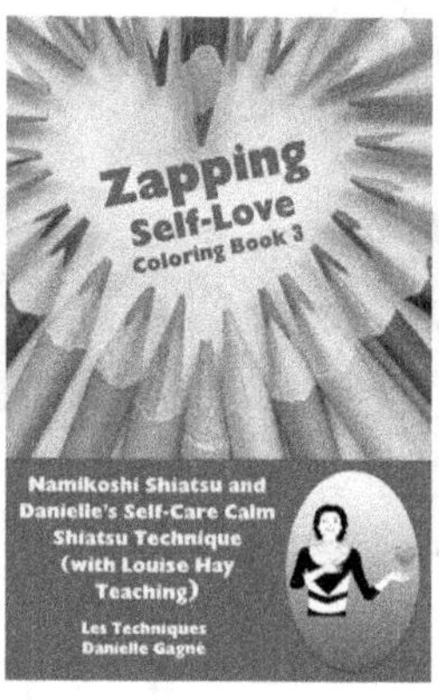
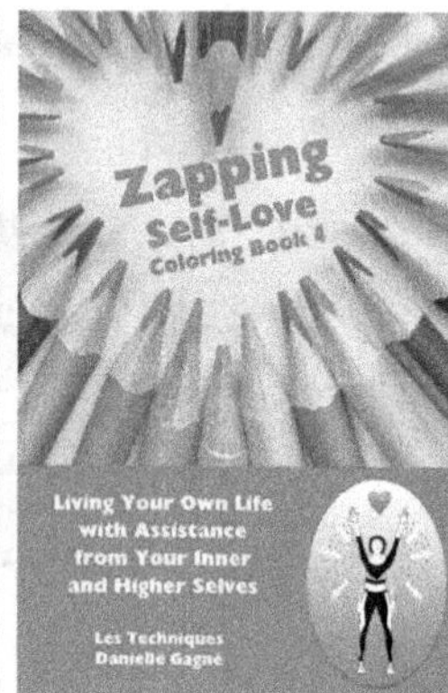
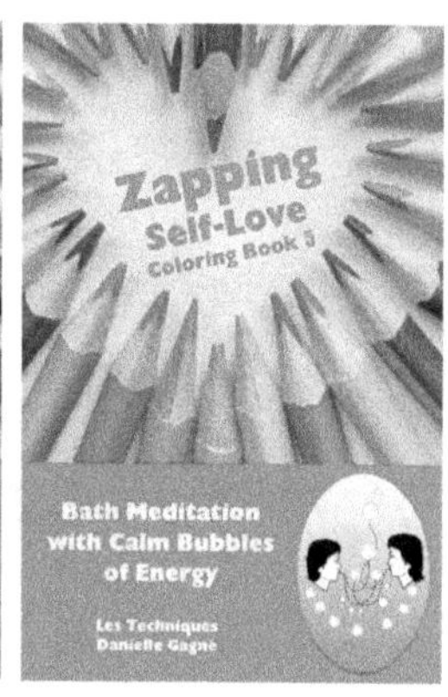

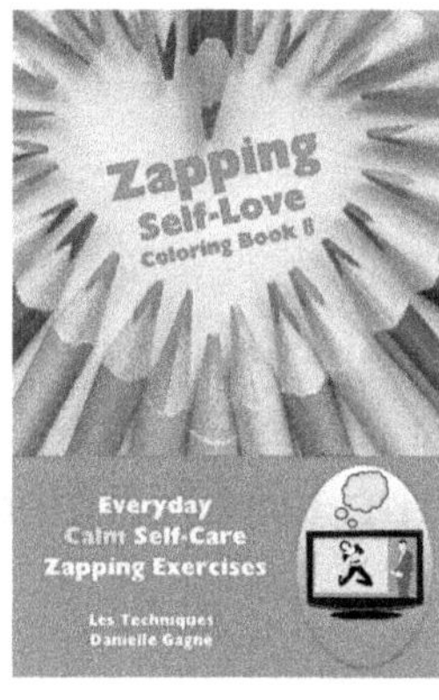
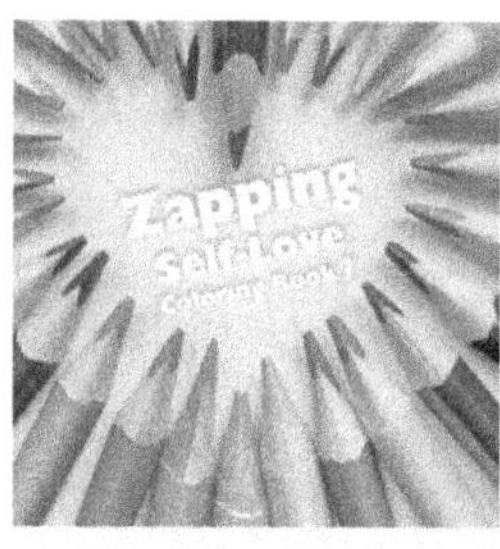
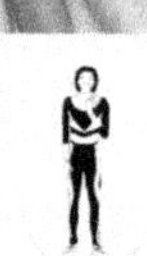
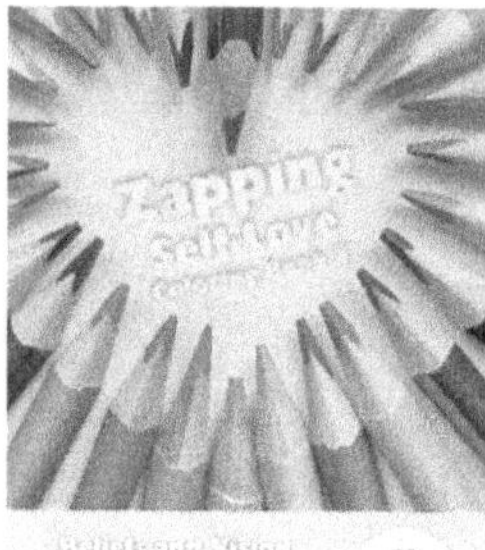
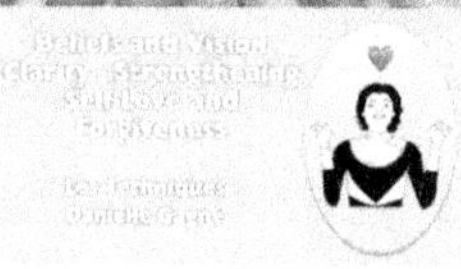
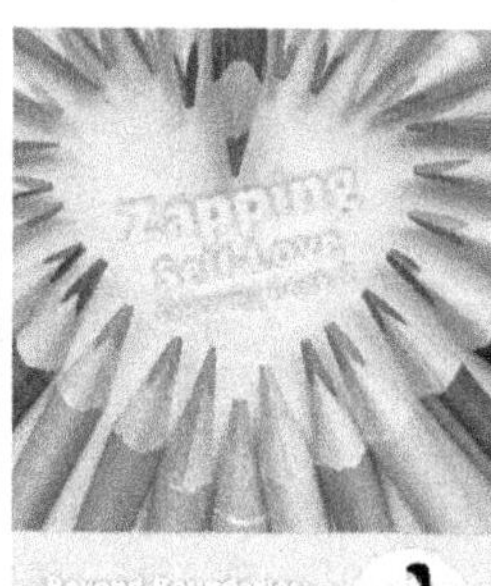
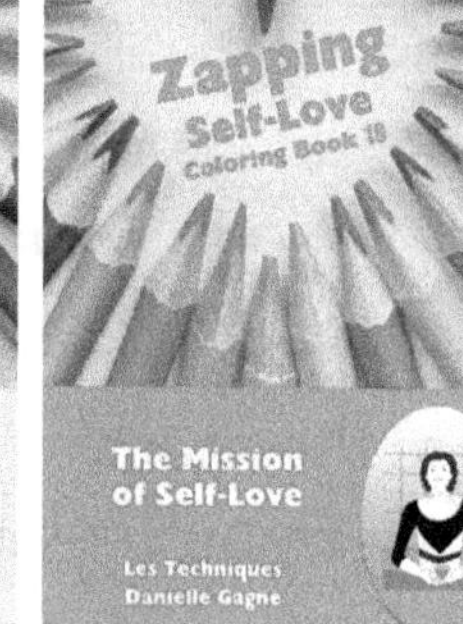

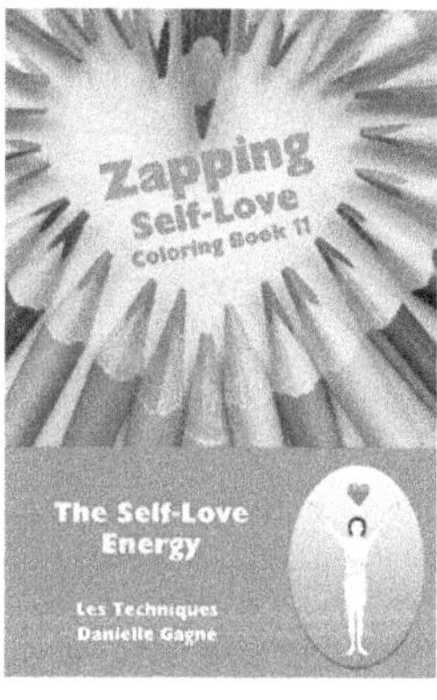
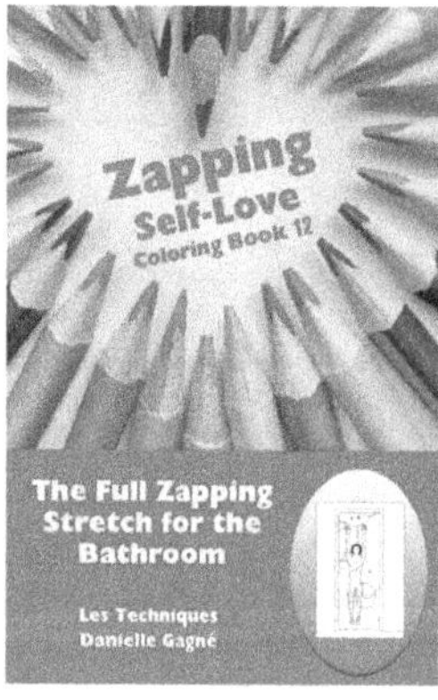
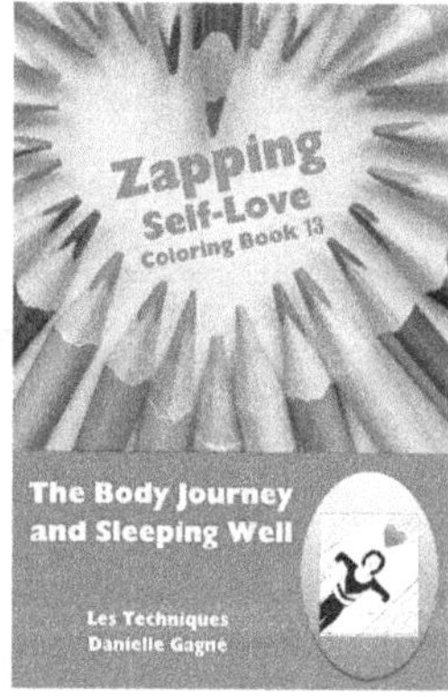
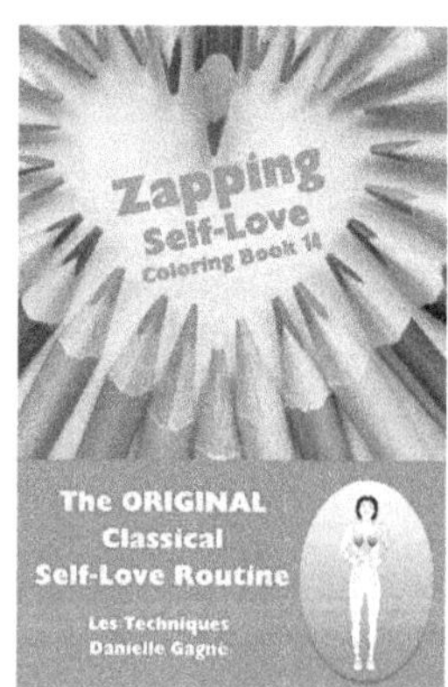

24